Contents

I0435622

STOP! Read This Section Before You Read The Rest of This Book.

This is a no fluff book that has been condensed down to the essential secrets of weight loss for busy parents like you. **I know you don't have a lot of time to read for hours at a time, and promise you that you can read it in less than 2 hours, while sitting in bed on Saturday morning drinking your coffee.** You won't find 100 pages of exercises, cover models and recipes, those are a dime a dozen in my opinion. Who has a ton of time to read a big thick book when you have tons of kids activities, honey do lists and work to do? Plus, if you are like me, you probably have a few 300 and 400 page "weight loss" books lying around in your basement or library.

The goal of this book is to teach you how to replicate the best weight loss tactics my 20 plus years of scouring books, magazines, videos, and seminars have thought me. **You will need to spend about 2 hours reading my story** on how I ended up gaining a six pack of abs, dropping over 20 pounds and losing 8% body fat—all in less than six months, while juggling a family, running my own business and working 60 plus hours a week.

This is not a magical book that promises you to lose 50 lbs. in 2 weeks. If you do what I teach you in the book for 6 months, you will be amazed at your results.

The book also has an accompanying resource website with my latest updates to help you get into the best shape of your life. The resource website has the following:
- My special Excel and Google Sheets tracking application to show you at a glance if you are on track or not

- Special report what works now in weight loss
- Audio and videos, including me giving a presentation that you can download and play in your car or on your smartphone

DISCLAIMER: The information provided by this book or by the Author is not a substitute for a face-to-face consultation with your physician, and should not be construed as individual medical advice. If a condition persists, please contact your physician. The testimonials on this book are individual cases and do not guarantee that you will get the same results. This book is provided for personal and informational purposes only. This book is not to be construed as any attempt to either prescribe or practice medicine. Neither is the book to be understood as putting forth any cure for any type of acute or chronic health problem. You should always consult with a competent, fully licensed medical professional when making any decision regarding your health. The owners of this book will use reasonable efforts to include up-to-date and accurate information in this book, but make no representations, warranties, or assurances as to the accuracy, currency, or completeness of the information provided. The owners of this book shall not be liable for any damages or injury resulting from your access to, or inability to access, this book and related websites, or from your reliance upon any information provided on this book.

IMPORTANT COPYRIGHT AND LEGAL NOTICE:
You do NOT have permission to copy, re-distribute, resell, auction, or otherwise give away copies of **Beginner's Guide to Ultimate Weight Loss for Busy Parents**, whether in electronic or physical book format. And yes, international copyright laws also protect electronic book copies.

If you attempt to do any of the above methods of distributing this electronic book or book, you are in violation of international copyright laws and are subject to fines and imprisonment. Copyright infringement is a serious crime with fines starting at $100,000 and up, including potential imprisonment upon conviction.

Acknowledgements

To God for all the blessings you have bestowed upon me

To my wife Mondi for being the best wife, friend and supporter a man could ever be blessed with.

To my two boys Sekayi and Farai, I love you so much.

To my Mom for always being there for me and teaching me the meaning of sacrifice and love.

To Shawn and Roxanne for being the best siblings in the world.

**Free Success Toolkit Included
Thank You for Purchasing the
Beginners Guide to Ultimate Weight Loss for Busy
Parents 1st Edition!**

Get a stream of updates and valuable resources (a very conservative value of $50) that will help you lose weight and stay healthy, track your new habits, stay focused, and help you become and stay healthy.

Here's what you get:
- My special Excel and Google Sheets tracking application
- Special reports, audio and videos, including me giving a presentation of what works now in weight loss
- Links to dozens of resources and tips for getting all your weight loss goals, which exercise programs I like, which nutrition programs I like

**Go to:
quickweightlossinsiders.com/book-supplement**

Introduction: You Can Look Your Absolute Best

Hi there; thanks for taking the time to pick up my book. My name is Andre Fraser, and I want to share my story on how I ended up gaining a six pack of abs, dropping 20 pounds and losing 8% body fat—all in less than six months!

I am 44 years old, the father of two boys and married to the love of my life. For the last 22 years, I've struggled with trying to get the perfect body. I must have tried a million different exercise plans, diets, etc. You name it, and I've tried it, from fat burners like Xenadrine to HotRox and more. I tried some extreme diets too, such as the velocity diet, when I went for four weeks with only four solid meals and spent the rest of the time drinking liquid protein shakes with flax seeds. I swear that I hallucinated a few times during this diet. Talk about being a grouchy person for four weeks! I even bought an electric Ab belt from one of those late night infomercials that was supposed to stimulate your mid-section so that you would have a six pack of abs without going to the gym. That lasted all of about 10 minutes. My stomach itched like crazy with the belt. What a joke! So now that I'm 44, I've finally been able to achieve my dream of looking like a mini-superhero. It's a long journey, and I learned a lot along the way. There were several products that I tried on my journey of finally get where I am today.

Major secret: Getting and keeping a six pack of abs is very simple. The fitness media wants you to believe that the latest diet fad or the latest exercise fad is going to help you get into shape and loose those love handles, cellulite and butt dimples. What they don't want you to know, is that the fitness media has been completely designed to deceive you and keep you confused. I learned this the hard way. Heck, it took me 20 years of trial and error to get here. I spent thousand dollars trying all the different weight loss fads, popular magazine subscriptions, such as Men's Health, Men's Fitness, Muscle & Fitness; you name it, and I bought them. I even had Flex magazine, that published an article saying that you to eat 10,000 calories per day to try and get bigger. You don't have to do anything extreme like signing up for a half marathon or a triathlon. I know all about extreme endurance, all in the name of getting in shape.

I've run half-marathons. I've done century rides (100-mile bike rides). I've done 150-mile rides in two days. Even with all of these activities, I still had soft, pudgy love handles. So my quest continued, and I finally cracked the code. I'd love to share my story with you and tell you the tools that I used to get here. I'll tell you what, the secret is not in doing more cardio. It's in not starving yourself and being unhappy eating chicken breasts and broccoli 24 hours per day. The system that I learned and the process that I used, well, I could eat my own home-created pizza, and I eat a lot of great spicy foods too. I love chicken and curries; yes, all the different things that we can think about, I get to eat.

Understanding how your body works is key. There's also a huge psychological component that most training programs and personal trainers don't take into consideration. As a business owner, I'm on-call 24 hours per day. I've got to be in the office. I've got to answer calls from my contractors. I've got to make collection calls. My day is booked solid. And then on top of all this, I've got two wonderful boys that I love very much, and I want to spend time with them. So how do you balance all of these pieces and still find time to get to the gym while still eating properly and preparing your own food? And on top of that, I've got a beautiful wife and we love to spend quality time together. So how do you go about doing all those things?

Now that I think about it, I even tried doing mixed martial arts, jujitsu, Muay Thai, judo…you name it, and I've done it. I've been punched in the face in hopes of getting leaner. Don't get me wrong, I did get some results. You're not going to get the sculpted bodies that you see on the magazine cover or on television by walking for one minute per day. There are a whole lot of different small things that you'll need to learn.

I've put together this book to outline a real and effective process for you. I also created a spreadsheet to allow you to hold yourself accountable, because that's going to be a huge factor in getting and staying lean and fit. There will be a point when you lose some weight initially from going to the gym. However, if you don't know what you're doing, that weight loss will plateau, and you will get frustrated. You will have to figure out how to get past those plateaus and remain encouraged, so you can keep improving.

I'm a busy father of two and a very happy husband with a very a happy wife, because I spend time with them. On top of this, I run a successful technology company. Realistically, maintaining balance in my life takes a lot of structure, commitment and planning. It's not a fad that you can master in two weeks. But if you're willing to work hard for a better life, I can definitely show you how to get you in the best shape of your life.

I can't believe that I'm fitter, lighter, healthier and more attractive (according to my wife) than I was in college. But let's be real—it's not just about looking good. It's also about being healthy and being able to perform better. I ride my bike twice a week with a group of my friends. Before I took my health seriously, I was always the guy in the back of the pack, struggling to catch up and breathing heavy with burning legs. Now that I've learned to exercise and eat better, I'm finally the guy leading the pack with the best of the riders. There are some strategies that I'm going to share that you will need to follow. If you're looking for a quick overnight fix, then I suggest that you go and get liposuction, which will cost you five or six thousand dollars. In six months, you'll be just as lumpy and bumpy as before, because your behavior has not changed.

I'll show you how to change your behavior and learn what you need to do in the gym. I'll even share some videos that I've used to work out and tell you about what I eat. I'll show you photos of the foods I eat too, so you'll have a great example of what to do in the kitchen, because that's a major part of being fit.

Chapter 1: Developing Your Winning Mindset

Let's talk a bit more about your mindset and fat loss, and I cannot stress how important this is. In my journey to get really lean, I used to spend lots of time reading Men's Health and Muscle & Fitness. And it was just all so confusing with conflicting information. I would try one program recommended by Men's Health, and initially, I would get some success, but after a while, I would get stuck and I wouldn't lose any more weight. You know, one day I would decide, "Okay, I'm so busy. I'm not getting results anyway, so I'm not going to go to the gym."

And then it would be two days and then three days, and then you know, in a month I may get to the gym five times for that month, but I still follow that same routine. You know, I was going to the gym, so why was I not getting all the results that I wanted? And once I realized that you have to track how many times you go to the gym and really stick to the habit, I realized that you really need to be close to 85% compliant. So if you think about it, five hours a week… that's close to 20 hours a month that you need to put into your schedule and get to the gym. Sometimes that could be tough with a busy life, but you really need to make it a priority if you want to get fit, healthy and perform better. At a certain point, you're going to reach a plateau.

Initially, when you start working out and eating differently, you're going to lose a lot of weight, especially if you have a lot of weight to lose. I didn't have a ton of weight to lose, you know, maybe 25 lbs. I initially thought that I just needed to lose 10 lbs., because I could see part of my ass outside of my pants. But it really turns out that I needed to lose 20 lbs. to look like I was in good shape. And that comes with its own issues, because it gets into your securities as a man. In society, we thought that bigger was better, so once you start losing the fat, your muscles don't look as big when you're wearing clothes. Before, you had a bunch of fat pushing up the muscles so you may have looked bigger, but you know, you never took your shirt off because you still had those love handles. Once you start losing weight, your face is going to look thinner and people are going to ask you, "Are you okay? Are you sick?", because everybody's so overweight that it's now become normal to think that people who are losing weight either have some kind of disease or they must be sick.

We are meant to have slim faces and we are meant to be lean and look athletic. We are not meant to be walking around with love handles, triple rolls of belly fat, back fat and flabby arms. It's not good for you, and it's not healthy for you. One of my biggest motivations was to avoid as many diseases as possible. High blood pressure and cancer are part of my family's medical history. I did not want to get sick one day and realize, "You know what? If I had cut down on sodas, juices and sweets, I would not have diabetes," or "If I had taken the time to exercise, eat healthy and monitor my blood pressure, maybe I would not have had a stroke."

There are things you can control and things you can't control, but I wanted to make sure that I did control the things that I could. So I really took it seriously. You know, I have two young sons that I want to be there for. I want to be healthy. Being healthy and strong means that when my boys want me to lift them up, I can do it without keeling over or being out of breath.

While you cannot always control how fast your body is going to lose weight, you can control your behavior. And your behavior to lose weight would be to follow the habits that I laid out earlier. It's all in eating lots of vegetables, eating complex carbs after exercise, and getting to the gym four or five times a week. These are things that you can control, and if you do these things, you will get the results. Sometimes your body is going to not shift, and your weight is not going to drop. If you've been going to the gym for five or six weeks where you are losing 1 or 2 lbs. per week, and all of a sudden you're no longer losing weight, you really just need to keep going and not give up.

It's like an egg. One of my mentors talked about this concept before. When you look at an egg, the egg doesn't bring forth a chicken on the first day, but there are a lot of things going on and changing on the inside of the egg. This is what happens to your body when you go to the gym and eat properly. There are lots of changes going on in the inside that may necessarily show up as a tangible drop in weight or an inch loss on your hips or your waist. But then one day, bam! That egg breaks open and you have this chicken. And that's what's going to happen. Some weeks you'll be like an egg and you'll keep going to the gym, grinding it out and grinding it out again, but there's no change. This is about what happened for me. Then on a Saturday morning, which is my 'weigh in morning,' I would get up, go to the bathroom and get on the scale, and I would've dropped 2 lbs. Then I would get my tape measurer out, because I measure every week, and I would've dropped a half inch on my waist. So there's no rhyme or reason as to how this happens, but I do know that if you are consistent with the habits and working out while eating properly, then you will drop the weight.

Learning how to change your current mindset is where the people are who get really fit and lean, and then there's the people who are just trying to get fit only; that's where I think our mindset separates us from getting there. What I mean by mindset is the way you react to different situations, or the way you set goals about what you want.

For years, I always knew that I wished I had a six pack of abs. I wished that I could get really lean and look like a superhero. That was always my goal, right? Every guy wants to have the nice, ripped, washboard abs, and women want to have that nice, goddess-looking shape. No wiggly underarms as they call them, and no extra piece of back fat, while guys just want to have bigger biceps, a bigger chest, and a washboard of abs.

When I started really looking at how I had set goals and how I tried to accomplish them, I realized that there was a big disconnect. Before, I would just wish. It really was a wish, and I would say, "Okay, this summer I'm going to the beach, so I want to get in shape." I would go to the gym maybe three times a week and just muck around in there and do some cardio, lots of cardio really. I would run every day, and I would initially lose some weight. I'd get stuck, and the first thing I would say is, "Argh! This doesn't work!" What happened the last time around is that I really had to change my feelings associated with going to the gym, how I felt when at the gym, and I had to start eating properly. I started associating pain with not being in sync with my goals; that is, I made it very painful if I did not achieve my goal of getting to 8% body fat.

So you know, it's tough sometimes, but you have to realize that you have to stick to it. Give it time. If that doesn't work, then it may be time to consult with the nutritionist to change one thing at a time. Don't just change your workout and change your eating habits at the same time if you're working with professional assistance, because then you won't know what causes weight drops. When you need extra help, really concentrate on changing one thing at a time.

There's several really good books on eating and exercise, so just check in my resource section.

Visit my resource page for up to date information and recommendations:
quickweightlossinsiders.com/book-supplement

I've got links for you there to find out more. Off the top of my head, John Berardi's "Precision Nutrition" has got a really good breakdown of eating habits. "The Truth about Abs" by Mike Geary goes into eating properly and describes some of the foods that are bad for you. There's also another good book called, "Burn the Fat, Feed the Muscle. "I also highly recommend reading a few books that will help you with changing your mindset about food, such as "The Omnivore's Dilemma" by Pollan and "I'm With Fatty" by Edward Ugel.

Chapter 2: How I Found a Real Mindset Shift for Reaching Fitness Goals

Initially, I was going to go for a certain weight, but weight measurements are not always the best indicator of your fitness. It's really all about your body composition and how much body fat you have. I started out at 16% body fat, and in six months, I was down to 8% body fat. I started out at 185 pounds, and in six months, I was down to 162 pounds. The first step in making a goal more realistic was in how I wrote it down, and every day I looked at it. There's a lot of books about goal setting. I'm not going to go through how to set goals here, but the major difference is to figure out what you need to do and do it. Posted on my computer, I had written a little note that read, "I'm going to do my best and get the best body composition I've ever had in my life." That was one thing, but the key here is I made a bet with my friends. I said, "Look, if I don't get down to 8% body fat in six months, I'm going to eat a can of Alpo dog food with raw eggs." Now that is just not a very good combination, but you know, now I had my ego on the line. I had people who knew that I was working toward my lean body composition goal. On days that I did not feel like going to the gym, I thought about, "Man, if I made a commitment to eat a can of dog food, which I do not want to eat, mixed with eggs to make it even worse, it's not going to taste really good. I'm going to get sick!" So you best believe that I busted my butt every day in the gym—that was the key ingredient.

Before my mindset change, when I worked out and I was on a so-called 'diet,' I tried to be very restrictive with what I ate. I went as far as trying not to go out to dinner at a restaurant. I would eat really, really bland food, but I learned how to adjust to life, because we all have children, and we all have people with whom we want to spend time. And you can't be fit at the expense of your family. You've got to go work 8 to 10 hours a day. You've got to spend some time with your wife; you've got spend time with the kids. You'll be spending time with those who are dear to you… So where exactly do you fit in your gym time?

My mindset changed to, "Look, I'm going to get up at five o'clock every morning and go to the gym. And if I can't get up at five o'clock, then I'm going to schedule a meeting with myself to go to the gym at lunchtime. And I will also track every time that I go to the gym, how many times I went, and how many times I missed it. After all, if you don't track it, then you're not going to follow through. You know, in a month or two months, you wouldn't know if you're meeting all your smaller goals.

And then of course, there's a time when your wife or other close family wants to spend some time with you, but it's time for you to go to the gym. Do you tell her, "Hey, I can't spend time with you. I've got to go to the gym"…? Or do you say, "Look, I'm flexible. Missing one workout or shifting my workout time is not going to change the world." If you think about it in the scope of six months to a year, or in terms of life, you then realize that it's a small price to pay and you'll have a happy wife, which in turn means you've got more time to go work out.

Bottom line, a happy spouse means that you can leave the house. So, the successful mindset so far is in being flexible and in making not reaching your goals painful. I had one friend who goes far as pledging to give $500 dollars to a charity that he totally despises. He has someone hold the money for him, so if he did not make that goal, then, guess what? He would literally have to give that money to a charity that—I think it was an abortion clinic, and he's pro-life so giving a donation to an abortion clinic would have been awful for him. It was really important to him to not support that charity, so he worked his butt off to make sure that it didn't happen. <u>The key point is to make it really, really, really hard and painful for you to not get to your goal. Knowing that you will face some real pain or misery if you do not get to that goal is huge.</u>

Now in terms of mindset shifts, maybe some of you are already really good at goal setting, but for me, I did not really understand the way that I should be setting new lifestyle goals. Coming into a new mindset for me meant that it was no longer just having the big 'pie in the sky' goal of six-pack abs, but it was really about developing new habits, that is, new ways of working toward that goal. In order for me to get to the six pack of abs, I needed to learn how to break this big, lofty goal into smaller habits. So I developed new habits. One of my habits was to get to the gym five days a week. So you know, I was going five days a week with an hour minimum.

Monday, Tuesday, Thursday, Friday and Saturday were the days that I spent in the gym. And that really helped, because I created a spreadsheet to track my habits for the entire month: did I go the gym or did I miss my workout. At the end of the month, I would know that of all the times I was scheduled to go to the gym, I got there 85% of the time, or I got there 50% of the time. This was a new way of looking at my workouts and tracking my weight loss goals.

It's also a good way to troubleshoot. If I'm not losing weight or I'm not losing any inches, then I could look at my compliance on my spreadsheet and say, "Okay. Well, you didn't go to the gym for the entire week. How are you going to lose weight?" By being able to track new habits of going to the gym and eating properly (which I will cover later, the eating habits that you need to really incorporate into your life), getting results that you want will become very real.

Let's talk about the key habits that are important for losing weight. First, you need to get to the gym. You need go to the gym for five hours a week and then track how often you actually get to the gym. I have a spreadsheet on my resource page where you'll find a link to my Google Docs Tracking Application. I will also make it available in Excel Format too.
Visit my resource page for up to date information and recommendations:
quickweightlossinsiders.com/book-supplement

Download this spreadsheet to use for tracking your habits. Track how many times you've been to the gym, your weight, and other things related to your fitness progress. It's just really nice to see a graphical representation. For starters, take your weight first thing tomorrow morning, and then measure your waist at your belly button. You need to keep track of these measurements every week as you practice this new habit.

Key habit: get to the gym four to five hours each week. And not just going to the gym, but working really hard, you know. Not strolling on tread mill, not just chatting with people, but really getting in there and kicking some ass. This applies to women too. Don't go on all the fancy machines. Just pick up a really good workout plan. I'm not going to cover work out plans here. I use several programs. I use P90X, I use the TRX rowing machine, and I also use a lot of free weights.

So there you have it: habit No. 1, get to the gym four to five hours each week. Habit No. 2, eat until you're 80% full. You should always be slightly hungry. Not starving, but slightly hungry. If you're not at this state, then you're overeating. I'll cover this later when we talk about the Okinawa diet named Hara Hachi Bu.

The third habit is eating veggies: one to two servings of veggies with every meal, and you could also add in some fruits. One serving of veggies is half a cup of vegetables.

The fourth habit is to only eat complex carbohydrates. Only eat the starchy carbohydrates after a very good work out; you know, you have to earn it. I made the game that if I wanted to go to dinner, I knew that I would want some starch and wasn't going to eat very well. I would work out for about 30 minutes to an hour. I would time my workout to happen right before I left home to go the gym, because I knew that I had a two-to-three-hour window to eat.

The fifth habit is to minimize the number of carb-loaded drinks that you consume. If it doesn't have zero carbs in it, I would not drink it. You know, orange juice, apple juice—all the different juices that are out there are not the best for you when you're trying to lose weight. They are packed with a lot of sugar, which in turn is really carbohydrates. But what that sugar does is... Actually, it's the level, but you know, I'm not a registered dietician. I just know that I've helped many of my friends to lose weight by just having them stop drinking Coke or Sprite, or whatever was their favorite soda or juice, and told them to just drink water.

Sometimes, drinking water can be hard initially. When you go cold turkey, drinking those sweet beverages is almost like a drug. You know, Gatorade is another slipper. Gatorade has a lot of high-fructose corn syrup, which is essentially sugar. So stay away from the Gatorade, your apple juice, and your orange juice. Drink lots of water. Try to drink two liters of water each day, which brings us to my next habit.

Drink two liters of water each day. Start off with maybe one liter and space this out through the day, and then build up to two liters. This will help flush your system and keep you from feeling hungry. A lot of times when you're hungry, you're really thirsty (in my experience).

To recap, we have you eating veggies with every meal, eating no complex carbs unless after a workout, and training five hours each week really hard. Another thing that you can do to really help with your intensity level in the gym is to look at some of the body-building stars' movies. Arnold Schwarzenegger has a movie that's called "Pumping Iron," and he really he shows you how hard those guys work to get the bodies that they wanted.

When you finish working out in the gym, you should be covered in sweat. For women, this is going to be hard on your hair, but maybe you can do it up early in the morning. I noticed several hair covers that you can use to help keep your hair from getting messy, but regardless, you're really going to have to work hard in the gym.

When I was going through my fat loss and getting really lean, it took a mindset change for me to eat vegetables at breakfast. For my entire life, I was trained that you ate bread with breakfast and rice with every other meal. Well, given the average sedentary lifestyle, we have to be a little more realistic. For many of us, the most exercise we get is walking to our car or walking up the stairs. If you eat a lot of complex carbohydrates without getting the appropriate amount of exercise, then your body doesn't process all of those complex carbohydrates and it turns into fat.

Remember, you need two vegetables and one fruit each day. So what I do is in the morning is to make an egg omelet with some spinach, onions, and mushrooms, and that takes care of my vegetable intake. For lunch, I may have an apple with a bowl of spinach, or I may make a nice stir-fry of peppers. When I talk about vegetables, the best ones to serve are all of the nice, green, orange, and red style of peppers, and broccoli, cauliflower, and carrots too.

The whole concept or reason behind eating vegetables is, of course, that all the vitamins and minerals that you will get from eating them. Eating a bowl of spinach and eating a bowl of rice gives you a totally different level of nutrition. Rice has a lot more carbs per square inch than a bowl of spinach. The basic rule is to eat more vegetables and only eat complex carbohydrates after you have worked out.

Chapter 3: Reality

As you can see from the photos that I'm attaching, this is not some smoke-and-mirrors overnight Photoshop job. This is me in August of 2010, weighing 185 pounds with 16% body fat. You see my love handles. This is me now. I took these pictures in January, and I'm 161 pounds with 8% body fat. Maybe I'm more around 5–6% body fat, but that's up for debate. The most important thing is I look a lot happier. I look younger. I feel better. You can too. I will show you how to also do this. I'm the regular guy that's walking down the street. I'm not a fitness model. I don't spend 20 hours in a gym every week. I don't starve myself. I still go out to eat. I still have fun with my friends. And I still have an alcoholic beverage from time to time.

It's not about killing yourself or restricting yourself to some wacky diet. It's not some kind of Jenny Craig or Weight Watchers thing, where you're eating food out of a cardboard box. It's really a way, if I had to summarize the approach, it's a happier way of learning how to BE fit, and just as importantly—learning how to STAY fit. Once you have met your fitness goals (fitting into an old pair of jeans, wearing a swimsuit in public, having an 8-pack of abs, etc.), how do you maintain that fitness level and positive mindset for years to come? I've cracked the code, and I want to share this insider knowledge with you!

One of the first things that I had to learn in my fitness journey is that traditional cardio (e.g., bike riding, walking and running) was just not very effective at getting fit and keeping a six pack of abs. This was one of the hardest things for me to accept. Think of all of your friends who want to get in shape; the first thing they do is they sign up for a big-ass endurance event. They sign up for the AIDS Ride, the Marine Corp Marathon, or whatever it is that they think is going to make them get in shape.

And it's not they do not get in shape, they do get some results. You may see them lose some weight if they were overweight or had a gut. If this is the way that you try getting into shape, then your stomach will go down a little bit, and your friends may notice that you lost a little weight. I ran several long races, and I also ran the Baltimore Half Marathon. I did several Century Rides, and still, I had love handles. WTF? Yes, my heart felt better and I looked a little thinner, but I didn't have the look that I wanted.

What I found out is that doing traditional cardio of going to the gym, riding or running four or five days per week, or how many times per week that you want, will get you looking a little slimmer, but you still have a gut. Think about it for a second. When you see most people running on a trail or riding a bicycle, most of them, if you see them up close, will have a gut. You never see the guys take off their shirts to run on the trail or the women wearing a crop top to show their stomachs. For women, they struggle to lose weight and still have big hips, or they have back 'love handles' as I call them, in that extra flesh right below their armpit. And of course, the wiggles when they wave, maybe you have the triceps hanging down that are really loose. They look like flags flapping in the wind.

Finding Your Fitness Mentor

Finding a fitness mentor is very important. There's a couple of reasons and advantages that I see—and it's about connecting with people. For one, it helps you stay motivated. There's an older gentleman that I know, and his name is Don. He's 55 years old, but he's one of the fittest people that I know. Whenever I work out with him, I would have to push myself to try to keep up with him, and that kept me going back to the gym. It made the gym fun. You learn a lot of different things when you work out with other people. Another guy, Courtney, taught me about eating more fats in my diet, because it's not about cutting fat out of your diet, it's really about having a balanced nutrition. We need fat to build up the testosterone level to build more muscle. More muscles burn more fat. Interesting, right?

By having a mentor, you can ask questions. I also had a few people that I worked out with; on the days that I did not feel like getting up or going to the gym, in the back of my mind I'm saying, "Oh, Andre, you've got to go to the gym because Stacey's going to be there. Richard is going to be there. How is it going to look if they show up in the gym and you're at home, sleeping in your bed?" You know, that time in the morning when you just wake up and it's early or you're tired? You feel like, "I really don't feel like going to the gym today."

But once you get to the gym, it just feels so much better. You have more energy; you feel good. You're sweating. You're making your body stronger. I loved it. And of course, there's a side effect that my wife thinks is so attractive, so you know, that leads to another set of benefits that I won't talk about in this book, wink, wink.

Getting a fitness mentor is good because you can learn different things and sometimes you can get them to look at your technique and correct it, if you are doing something wrong. My fitness mentor helped me realize that an exercise I had thought was an abs exercise was really a hip exercise! Learning new things and pushing yourself is key. Also try to be a mentor to people who are not as fit as you are. And don't be rude about it. If this is somebody who's very overweight and trying to do sit-ups, you don't say, "That's not going to work, Lard Ass." Instead you could say, "Hey, why don't you come work out with me? Let me show you a different way of getting to that six pack of abs," or just talk about what are they working on, what they're trying to achieve and if it is working for them.

As my mentor would say, "How is that working for you?" When you say this, just think that this person is doing sit-ups, and you ask him how long he have been doing the sit-ups for and say, "Hey. So how is that working for you?" It makes them think. It made me think when I was doing a whole lot of cardio, thinking that this was the way to get lean and fit with a bit of six pack coming too, but it wasn't working. But I kept doing it, because that's what the fitness media told me was going to happen.

Once I really got feed up, I took the chance and said, "Look, I'm going to listen and I'm going to work hard in the gym... and cut back on my cardio." Then the results came in. So really, reach out to people, help them, and have fun. I feel great when I help people. Nothing makes me feel better than someone coming back six months later saying, "You know, because of you I lost 25 lbs. after I stopped drinking soda," or "Hey, I stopped doing crunches and did more dead-lifts, or bench press, or squats, and now look at me. My arms are bigger, my back is broader or my waist is leaner." So now you know to pay it forward. Having a mentor and being a mentor is really, really good for keeping you lean and fit.

Chapter 4: Expecting Miracles by 'Working Out'

If you go to the gym and you observe people during lunch or dinner, all of the machines being worked on are cardio machines. You have the tread mills. You have the elliptical machines. You have the Stair Master and everyone is climbing. It is shocking that everyone is out of shape. Now, you really have to think about it: Why is that? Everyone has this whole concept of the fat-burning zone, so it means that you're supposed to go and run on the tread mill or get your heart rate up to a certain level, and then you'll burn fat.

The unfortunate thing about this approach to getting fit is that you don't lose weight or burn fat as soon as you step on the machine. The fat-burning zone on the machine only kicks in after you have finished the warm-up portion. So it takes you about 10 to 15 minutes to warm up. It takes about 10 minutes to get in the fat-burning zone and 10 minutes to cool down. And there you have 30 to 35 minutes, which is what most people do in a gym. As a matter of fact, most gyms limit you to 30 minutes on the treadmill or whatever the newest "fancy fat-burning machine" craze is. "Cardio" is an abused term. It's really an abused exercise habit. And it's really abused because most people in the gym think that it's the way to a trimmer you. If you stop and think about it, when you look at long-distance runners or marathon runners, they look very slim but they're not necessarily muscular. When you look at a sprinter, they are very muscular and more balanced. Really, we mostly want to look like a sprinter versus a marathon runner or an endurance athlete. So one of the things that I had to change was to stop running, stop cycling, and change the type of cardio exercise I did.

What I want to do is explain to you is the correct use of cardio with how you're eating. If you're going to do any kind of activity, your first bet should be that your nutrition is your number one priority. So, what you put into your mouth should always be the first thing you'll consider. So that's number one. Number two is also about nutrition again. So that's really important. You really cannot outrun, outride, out-lift, out-cardio, a very bad diet. There's no way to do that, so why run for half-an-hour and burn maybe just 100 calories. Yes, you may burn 60 to maybe even 200 calories, but then you go and eat a slice of pizza—or two or three slices of pizza, which may end up being 600 or 700 calories. So really, you've just defeated the whole purpose of exercising and doing cardio.

Setting Up Actionable, Achievable Fitness Goals

This section is on how you go about implementing all of these things that I cover in this book. And really, the secret is not to jump and try to do everything the same week or try to change your eating and your diet all at once. It's just way too much, too soon, and you will get frustrated and run out of steam.

A lot of people buy a new home-study course that comes with 20 CDs and 5 DVDs, and 20 big binders; you start off really nice. "Oh, yes! This is great!" For about three days, you'll read and listen to the DVDs, but then life takes over. After a while, you end up not doing anything. So what I recommend are a couple of things that I have included in my tracking spreadsheet. I want you to just really learn one thing at a time. It's one habit. So pick one thing. Make the commitment and say, "You know what? I'm going to eat one to two servings of veggies per meal." I want you to get about six servings of veggies in a day so you'll keep going and moving along on adding veggie servings, one at a time and at your own pace. It's really just to put a check mark in the sheet and to say, "Hey, I ate my veggies today."

At the end of the day, if you had six serving of veggies, that's great. That's all I want you to do. And then do this for three weeks until it becomes like second nature. Then try adding the next habit, "I'm going to go to the gym five hours a week." You try that. And every day that you go to the gym, you give yourself a star. Soon enough, this will become second nature. You will see that you've done your veggies, and you've done your workout.

Add one habit at a time. Don't try to do ten things at the same time. Just make sure to track it all and you will be surprised at how these things become second nature. You know, things like taking your fish oil and your multivitamins or taking your complex carbohydrates after meals. So just really practice adding your checkmarks and stars one at a time. Get your calendar out and mark it 'OK'. "Week No. 1 and No. 2—I'll do veggies. After that, I'll practice going to the gym.

You're building one habit on top of another habit. You're just not saying, "Okay. I'll eat veggies for two weeks" and then stop eating veggies before going on to working out for a couple weeks and then dropping that too. No, you're going to work out for two weeks—and make it a habit. Then you'll keep working out while longer. Then in another two weeks, you'll find that you're still eating your vegetables, and in two weeks after that, you add in your fish oil, so now you've now mastered three habits. Move on it step-by-step, and you will make those a life-long way of working out into getting and keeping your lean body.

I've actually started using this same method in my business and for achieving my other life goals. Whatever I want, I figure out which habits I need to develop, and next I'm working on those habits, one at a time. It's definitely made a difference, even in writing this book. I made the conclusion, "You know what? I'm going to start doing a chapter a day. Sometimes I do two chapters each day, but at least I made progress toward my larger goal of writing a book, and here it all is for you.

Chapter 5: Working Out: The Real Deal

But for this goal, if you want to look like a superhero, I want you to concentrate on getting to the gym, lifting really heavy weights, or working out at home and lifting really heavy weights also. I do recommend going to the gym. Why?

The type of cardio that I recommend is high intensity cardio. The secret is working really hard for maybe 20-30 minutes. Cycling or running as hard as I can for 100 meters, and walking for 200 meters. That's where you'll get the most return on your investment, because what this kind of elevated and aerobic exercise does is that it creates something called 'epoch.' This may not necessarily burn fat when you do it, but it elevates your metabolism and your heart rate, and your whole body goes into a fat-burning mode for almost 24 hours after. There are many studies that have shown this to happen.

Hey, we are not here to talk about studies, you're here to learn about what works. And what works is to go to a gym, bust your butt for 30 minutes, or go to a local high school track and do your best to work up a sweat. You know, you're going to work for this. So that's what I have to say for cardio. I'm going to put some links to some really good conditioning programs in the resource section, such as including Turbulence Training. The TRX training has several conditions, that is, systems and circuits that you can use to get in shape.

Visit my resource page for up to date information and recommendations:
quickweightlossinsiders.com/book-supplement

Another suggestion for effective cardio that I know, if I had to recommend cardio in the gym, is spinning class. That's an excellent class. It's 45–60 intense minutes that really gets the sweat out of you. And what else? Zumba class, that's possible. This is all definitely better than running on a treadmill at slow pace. If you think about what it means to run in a tread mill, it's kind of like hopping on one leg for 3,000 strides, and then on your other leg for 3,000 strides. Would you really do that?

Let's talk about what kind of exercise you should do. Should it be the latest and greatest Zumba class? Should it be P90X? In essence, when you break your five weekly exercise hours into what you should be doing, you really need to just concentrate more on working hard than worrying about any specific method. Work on really big compound movements when you exercise, things like pull-ups and dead-lifts. When I left the gym, I was pretty sore for a couple of days. I would do four days of lifting weights and one to two days of sprints on the bike or sprints on the treadmill, activities where I worked really hard and got my heart rate really high. Spinning class is really good for this, and maybe a Zumba class can be fit in here too. Some of you guys think that "it's just a Zumba class," but if you're working hard with a group, you're more likely to push yourself than if you're working alone.

I'm not going to give you one recommended workout

program, but I have several programs that I do recommend that are very thorough. If you are the kind of person who is able to work out at home, then I highly recommend the P90X program followed by Insanity. On the days that I could not get to the gym because of my schedule, I would turn on the TV and load up one of my P90X DVDs; you'll work out really hard for an hour with P90X. It's a thorough program, so I recommend P90X first because it combines weights with calisthenics, so you get a complete work out. The Insanity program is good because it's all body weight.

Visit my resource page for up to date information and recommendations:
quickweightlossinsiders.com/book-supplement

If you're like me and you like to be around a lot of people in the gym, then I recommend trying Alwyn Cosgrove's fitness conditioning too. I also like CrossFit for the days that I do high intensity training, when I may do lots of push-ups, lots of pull-ups, as much as I can do for 20 seconds and then rest, and then do a lot of box jumps, and these kinds of independent exercise things. And I like Monkey Bar Gym because they give you different conditioning workouts that you can do. But I don't do this too often. I just do Monkey Bar Gym or CrossFit—maybe once a week, because it's a different mindset. You can get yourself in shape at CrossFit, so I love their workouts. It's based on working really hard for 20 minutes or 10 minutes, or 15 minutes, or sometimes even an hour.

When you travel, the TRX rocks, because it's more like a band that you hang on your door, and you can leave it on your door at home to use when you're not traveling. You can even just go to a local playground and connect to the one with swings to get a really good workout from that.

Do you need some books to get you going? Books that I like include Mike Geary's "The Truth about Abs". He has a really good nutrition and training program. I also love "Turbulence Training" by Craig Ballantyne, who has really good programs on how to lose weight even if you're a busy person.

The whole intent here is that whether you go to the gym or you're working out at home, you want to push your body and get it into a metabolic state of burning fat. Instead of just burning fat in a supposedly "fat-loss zone" for 15 minutes, you're burning fat for 24 hours. It really does all work if you use it; all these workout tools can really push you hard and work you really hard. And of course, you can get a different workout each day so that you stay motivated.

Chapter 6: Eating Until You're Satisfied

This is such a major part of losing weight. For a long time, I was not in touch with my body, so I would tend to just eat. Even when I thought that I was eating really, really healthy food, I found out that I was eating close to nothing when it came to real nutrition. I would actually consume food every day that I did not need. The concept of eating until you're satisfied is based on the Okinawan diets. If you'll notice in Okinawa, most of the people are in shape, but the whole culture stops eating when they're about 80% full. For people outside of this culture, this habit takes some practice.

Ninety percent of the people eat all the food on their plate because their parents made them clean their plates before leaving the table.

In essence, if you were eating four to five small meals per day and finishing everything on your plate, then your objective here is to stop eating when you think you're about 80% full. Boy! This takes practice. If you feel hungry after stopping at 80%, then give yourself about 20 minutes before you eat some more food. A great place to start in estimating your 80% is with the amount of food that you currently eat and then just leave 20% on the plate. And in 20 minutes, if a bowl of broccoli or a bowl of carrots looks attractive to you, then more than likely, you're still hungry. So then you should eat a little bit more. The concept is that in two to three hours, you should be hungry again.

If you're starving two to three hours later, then this means that you did not eat enough, and you should increase the amount a little bit more. If you don't feel hungry two to three hours after you ate, then you had too much to eat. So it's a balancing act, but you can really get a feel for what your body needs. Studies have shown that your body does not signal your mind about fullness until 20 minutes after you're actually full.

Caveat: If you try to eat until you're full, then you've already overeaten. When I started practicing Hara Hachi Bu, as is practiced by the Okinawa people, I started losing one pound a week. Just like that. Before, my weight had stuck and I was exercising five hours a week. I was losing inches on my waist and different parts of my body, but my overall weight was not going down.

I started really listening to my body and listening to my hunger cues while asking questions like: Am I really hungry? Does a bowl of spinach look really good? Or is my mind playing tricks on me? I then started to see a massive change in the way my body responded. The weight just started coming off. You know, some weeks it would be two pounds, some weeks it would be one pound. But it's one of the key areas in learning to eat properly that will help you drop a lot of weight. That's it.

Let's review the key habits that are important for losing weight. One, you need to get to the gym. I went to the gym five hours a week. For four or five days, I got there, and I busted my butt. Really, go to the section of the gym that you need to pick up a really good work out plan.

Habit No. 2, eat until you're 80% full. You should always be slightly hungry. Not starving, but slightly hungry. If you're not in this state, then you're overeating. I covered that earlier with describing the Okinawa eating habits and their Hara Hachi Bu diets.

The third habit is eating veggies, and the fourth habit is to only eat complex carbohydrates. Your fifth habit will be to minimize the number of carb-loaded drinks that you're drinking right now and drink two liters of water each day instead.

Setting Up Your New Kitchen

Let's talk about your kitchen makeover. This is going to be key to your immediate and long-term success. Initially, when I started about 20 years ago with trying to get into good shape, I would go to the grocery store and buy all the regular things: chicken breast, broccoli and a few deserts. Of course, I'll come home with all the intentions of cooking everything I bought. Most times, however, I would put it off because prepping the vegetables took so long and it was just cumbersome.

At the recommendation of a few people, I did a full kitchen makeover starting from where I went into the pantry. I cleaned up the pantry and got rid of all the stored junk foods. If I really want to eat some cookies, I'll go to Subway and buy a cookie and eat it. But by keeping it all at home, eventually you're going to give in to the temptation of eating that junk food. I also started buying a lot more fruits and vegetables. I cleaned up the pantry, cleaned out the refrigerator, and I always try to keep the refrigerator freshly stocked with meats and vegetables. I also make it a point to have all of the great fruits that we all like to eat.

Additionally, I keep lots of freezer bags around. Whenever I cook a meal, I'll take one or two pieces and set them aside in a freezer bag. These are good for when I'm in a pinch and I don't feel like cooking, or in fact, when I'm just being lazy. I then have no excuse but just to take a piece of chicken stuffed with goat cheese and heat it up. This method of having food ready really minimizes the amount of time that you would want to eat junk food, because you have a ready supply of delicious food.

Now, let's talk about equipment. I had some cheap knives. I never thought there was a difference in having real knives, and I could not understand why people would spend so much money on getting knives. But I did upgrade the knives in my kitchen, and all of a sudden, it became so much easier to prepare vegetables and chop things up. In really redoing your workspace, you need to get some proper mixing bowls. I got a set of really nice mixing bowls from Costco and several cutting boards, because you want to have an area set up in your kitchen where you can cut up all your vegetables if you enjoy doing this kind of stuff, like I do. I got a pretty nice set of Gunter Wilehm, four blade knives that are very sharp. It's just fun cutting things up, and it's much easier prepping food.

Then I added a Teflon non-stick frying pan to my kitchen tool set; this was essential because I do a lot of food prep. The last thing you want to happen as you're making a really beautiful-looking omelet is that it sticks to bottom of the pan. Then you have to make it into a scrambled egg; bummer! So having a nice set of pots, you know, go spend the extra money. Go to Costco, where there's usually a lot of great deals on nice cookware. I also got a set of stainless steel pots and a pressure cooker. I love having my pressure cooker, which is like a hyperspace version of a slow cooker.

Normally, most people would spend 10 hours cooking in a slow cooker. For the pressure cooker, you can have a very tough cut of meat done to tender in about 45 minutes. You can get one of these pressure cookers from Fagor, Amazon, or Hex, which is a good place to start. Just read the instructions, which will tell you how long it takes to cook peas, lentils, meats and more.

Let's review what to change with your kitchen upgrade. Clean your pantry out. Clean your refrigerator out. Stock it with fruits and snacks. Keep lots of fruits in the house, so that when you're hungry, you can eat a piece of fruit versus eating a piece of tiramisu. Upgrade your knives. Get some nice pots, pans, mixing bowls and a blender.

Here's a funny story. For years I had a very cheap blender in my kitchen, and it was the worst thing for trying to make fruit smoothies. I would have a lot of frozen berries in there, and you could literally smell the smoke coming out of my blender. This is when you realize that you have a couple of options for replacement. Some people swear by the Vitamix, and some people swear by the Blendtec. I have a Vitamix. Before the

Vitamix, I had a Ninja 3 set of blades blender. I thought it was awesome, until one fatal day I walked into a Vitamix demo at Costco. My intent was to make fun of the people, but I some how ended up spending a little under $400. It is worth every penny. That's my story and I'm sticking to it. :-)

All of the guys that I hang out with online who have Vitamix love making soup with their blenders. So I'll include this in the resource page for you to take a look at as well as a few others I have had the opportunity to use.

Visit my resource page for up to date information and recommendations:
quickweightlossinsiders.com/book-supplement

What else? Add lots of spices. Eating bland food is just not a good way to sustain yourself and get lean. I love eating; I love spicy food; I love food with flavor, and I hate eating chicken breast with broccoli or steamed rice. It's just not what I want to do.

There's a lot of great cooking books, and you can make some excellent meals by reading about fine cooking. These cookbooks are a great place to find good recipes, but many times you will have to modify them to remove all the fats. A minimum amount of spice is all you really need to add the flavor, and you can drop the five tablespoons of butter. If a recipe calls five tablespoons of butter, then use half a tablespoon and you'll be fine.

Eating Out

Now, let's talk about eating out. When you start to work on becoming very lean, you're no longer going to spaz out and tell people, "I'm on a diet! I can't go to lunch. I can't go to dinner." There's no need for that. You just need to learn how to modify and bend the will of the restaurant's menu to your will. For example, don't eat any bread when you sit down for dinner.

Most restaurants serve portions that are two to three times what you would normally eat. When you get to the restaurant, drop the rice, drop the pastas, and substitute that with vegetables and lean meats. Most restaurants will allow you to say, "I would like a bowl of spinach," or "I would like mixed vegetables with no oil or butter," or "I just want plain vegetables with a little bit of garlic or onions." Stay away from anything that has a cream base such as Chicken Alfredo any meat with a creamy sauce. At the very least, have the waiter put the sauce on the side. There are a lot of hidden calories in the restaurant's food, especially in the rice and pastas. They put on a lot of butter and a lot of oil. Substituting the rice and pastas for vegetables will substantially reduce the amount of calories that you take in, which will go a long way toward you being a lean, mean, fighting machine.

The other thing is that if you're going to have a soup, go for a soup that has a broth base and is more watery. Skip the French onion soup, which is really just big globs of cheese—that's why it's very delicious. There may be 1,000 calories in that bowl, so it's not very healthy for you. Again, stay away from cheesy type style or cream-based style soup. If you're going to have a Crab Chowder, maybe there's very small bowl of it available. You could try to go for a taco soup for a change, or anything different that can keep you interested in what you are eating.

We have a natural tendency to eat what's placed in front of us, since our parents told us as children, "Oh, eat everything that's on your plate. Eat all your food or you can't leave the table!" As a kid, I prided myself on being the person who could put away a ton of food. It didn't matter if my stomach hurt, I would just keep eating and eating and eating. While we know that some people win eating competitions, it won't help with your love handles or your hips.

Normally, when I eat at a restaurant and my food comes to the table, I divide it into two portions and ask the waiter to package half of the food to go. I'll eat all of my vegetables, but I would pretty much take home half a portion of what I would have otherwise ate in one sitting before changing my mindset.

Conclusion: Keeping Your New Look for a Lifetime

It's all about maintenance. Once you get to the point where you're happy with the way you are in terms of your weight loss, this is where a lot of people have no idea about what to do next. After all, most of the books on fitness and health are really based around losing the fat. But what happens when you get to the end-point? You've lost the fat, and you feel great! Life is terrific, your health is exceptional and your blood pressure is down. You need to learn a few things to maintain fitness—you'll need to measure your body, which includes your chest, shoulders, hips, waist, thighs, calves and biceps, to make sure that your body stays within your ideal range.

You know, you can adjust your diet and exercise program if your weight starts going up again. You also need to learn what's called a 'trigger habit.' And for me, I found out that tiramisu or any kind of sweets is where I break down and can't stop eating. So, that's a trigger habit for me. For some people it's bread, and for others it's certain movies that trigger an emotional situation of too much eating. So once you learn your trigger habits, you really need to manage them properly, and you need to become more resilient.

I learned that I cannot keep any type of desserts in the house. In the past, I would have half a cake just sitting in the refrigerator and I would say, "No, I'm strong. I can resist it." But eventually, I would give into temptation, break down, and eat it.

So now, I recognized that tiramisu and sweets like that area trigger for me. I don't keep them around in the house. If I really want to have some tiramisu, then I will schedule it around the time after working out, go out with my wife, and I'll have a slice of tiramisu. I will also not abuse the fact that now I'm lean; I know this does not means that I can just eat what I want because I exercise. I found out the hard way that what I was doing was wrong: I would work out all week and be really good, and then on Friday nights, I would go to dinner and eat some Thai food with some wine and desert.

When I started counting up the amount of food that I had put into my system, eating Pad Thai with some dessert, two or three glasses of wine, and a soup, I found that was taking in 4,000 calories easily without even knowing it. I was thinking that, "Hey, I worked out all week so I can afford to eat crap on the weekends." But that's where you pretty much lost all the gains that you made, and you really can't out-work a bad diet. You can go to the gym five hours each week, but if you're not taking care of your diet and being really consistent with new habits of eating veggies, some dietary fats, and no starchy carbs before but only after a workout, then you're going to gain all the weight back. So it's really about changing your mindset to know that once you get to the way that you want to be, you cannot just abuse your new privilege.

Also, it's initially harder to wrap your mind around the fact that you're no longer losing weight, and you're no longer losing inches, but your body is the same day in and day out. So initially, it's hard; but after a while, it becomes a beautiful thing, because you realize that your body is happy, you're happier, you maintain your weight, and you enjoy the journey of going to the gym. Maybe it's time to pick up a new outdoor activity like cycling. I love cycling, so I spend one of my hours for my five exercise hours per week on my bicycle.

Once you get your routine down, then maybe you can slowly try to add about one complex carbohydrate meal into your diet and see if your body reacts to it in a bad way or in a good way. What we are talking about here is really a life-long experiment, a life-long journey of feeling good and looking great. Nothing beats being able to go to the men's store and buying that slim-fit shirt to show off your well-defined arms. Trust me, it's a great feeling, and you can do this too!

Visit my resource page for up to date information and recommendations:
quickweightlossinsiders.com/book-supplement